BEFORE YOU
TIE THE KNOT

Titles in the Angela Butts-Chester Library

Morning Tea

apart of : *Living With Grace A Collection of*
Purposeful Inspirations by Rev. Paula T. Webb

BEFORE YOU
TIE THE KNOT

Premarital Counseling workbook

for the DIY couple

ANGELA BUTTS-CHESTER

"Before You Tie The Knot"

Angela Chester Ministries

Long Beach, CA 90802

Scripture References

All scripture references are stated using the New International

Version (NIV), unless otherwise stated

ISBN: 978-0-557-02164-2

© Cover design – AMillion Graphix

© Cover photo – Eric Corbacho

Printed in the United States of America

This book is dedicated to every couple
who seeks to have a lasting loving bond
with their partner.
To have a marriage that will stand
the test of time.

May the Lord bless you and keep you.

ACKNOWLEDMENTS

I would like to thank the countless people that have allowed me to listen to their stories and learn from their "beauty parlor wisdom".

Always, grateful to my parents, for allowing me to be the person that God wants me to be. For being patient with me and allowing me to grow.

To my son – thank you for sitting with me as I typed. I loved our talks.

To my husband – thank you for understanding my late nights and having a pot of coffee ready every morning. You are the love of my life.

PREFACE

Congratulations on your engagement! You have waited for this moment your entire life and it has finally happened. I hope that it was exactly what you had imagined.

Getting engaged is a wonderful stage in a woman's life. It brings about an urgency that cannot be ignored. There is a need to plan every moment of the day for that one day – your wedding day. While, you must choose the correct China pattern, and no bride worth her veil would be caught without the perfect dress, don't forget to take a moment out to nurture your relationship just one more moment.

Some couples feel that going to premarital counseling is old fashion and out dated, but there's something to be said for proper planning. Counseling is not someone trying to tell you what to do and when to do it. It is a third set of eyes and ears to guide you along the touchy topics. That unbiased person who makes sure that no one hits below the belt. It is a time for open and honest discuss. Those sessions nor this workbook are used to break you apart from each other. Instead, it is used to show you those things that you may need to discuss further or quite possibly discuss for the very first time.

I know, many of you have already had the "big talk" with each other about all things important, but maybe, just maybe, you forgot to ask that <u>one</u> question. Maybe you were to shy to ask the other question – this workbook will do that for you. This workbook touches on all types of topics just enough for you get a very good idea of the other person's point of view. Some questions may even lead to other questions not listed here. Go for it – keep the conversation going. This is the person that you are about to marry. Let them know how you feel.

Now, does this mean that just because you disagreed about a certain something, that your fiancé will now come over to your point of view because you purchased this workbook – nope! But the fact that you've had the dialogue is a step in the right direction. I like to think of premarital counseling the proactive step to a positive marriage. It is better to go before than to have to go after. So enjoy your engagement. Don't work yourself into a tizzy if you can't find the perfect pair of white pumps. It will all turn out just fine.

May God bless your marriage. May patience, love, kindness and compassion dwell in your home.

Blessings to All,

Rev Angela Butts Chester

TABLE OF CONTENTS

TOPICS OF DISCUSSION

As you go through the workbook numerous topics are discussed with questions on each to follow. Some of you, may find the questions easy to answer, others may require some thought. While this workbook is not as extensive as in-house counseling by your local pastor, you will have an idea of the many issues that you will have to deal with within a marriage.

The following topics will be discussed:

- Relationship
  From how do you treat each other and what makes you tick. What are your desires for this relationship?

- Finances
  Have you decided how you will handle your money issues? Is she better or is he better at balancing the books?

- Home

Now that you have gotten your new place, have you decided on who will take care of the day to day routine?

- Housekeeping

  Will this be a "traditional" setting with male and female duties, or will you share in the chores?

- Children & Parenting

  To be or not to be parents – that is the question!

- Social Activities

  Will you still be apart of your social clubs, or join any? Will you attend a house of worship?

- Red Flags

  Do you know the signs of mental or physical abuse? Are you a victim?

If you find that you are having a hard time with the questions, seek local pastoral assistance. If you find that some of the red flag topics are a reflection of your relationship, please seek local professional assistance.

In this same way, husbands ought to love their wives as their own bodies.

He who loves his wife loves himself.

EPH 5:28

RELATIONSHIP

Everyone has a different idea of what makes up the ideal relationship. Have you discussed your needs and desires? How will being married affect those desires and needs?

One of the most important aspects of any relationship is the communication in that relationship. We must remember that our fiancé is not a mind reader, therefore, couldn't possibly know our every wish and desire until we articulate it. Use this section as a way to discuss those things that you may have not been able to articulate yourself.

As you answer the following questions be sure to answer honestly so that the other can learn from your answers.

1. Do you trust and love your fiancé?

   □ Yes □ No

2. Is your fiancé an honest and truthful person? □ Yes □ No

3. Do you feel your fiancé loves and trusts you? □ Yes □ No

4. How will you make day-to-day decisions once you are

   married?

   _____

   _____

   _____

5. How will you make major decisions once you are married?

   _____

   _____

   _____

   _____

   _____

6. Which word best describes your times when you don't see eye-to-eye *(circle)*:

   Debate Fight Argument Squabble

    Disagreement Misunderstanding

7. How would you handle/settle this "disagreement"?

_____

_____

_____

_____

_____

8. What do you do if you can't agree?

_____

_____

_____

9. Is it hard to say please, thank you and I'm sorry?

  □ Yes □ No

10. Will your parents be living with you?　　□ Yes　□ No

11. Will your fiancés parents be living with you? □ Yes　□ No

12. When you are not feeling well how much sympathy and attention do you feel you need?

_____

_____

_____

_____

13. How will you handle life insurance and estate planning issues?

_____

_____

_____

14. How would you handle end-of-life decisions?

_____

_____

15. How will you relate to in-laws, opposite-sex friends, ex-spouse or children from previous relationships after you are married?

_____

_____

_____

_____

_____

16. Do you believe your fiancé will be faithful? ☐ Yes ☐ No

17. Do you believe that you will be faithful to your fiancé?

    ☐ Yes ☐ No

18. Can you see yourselves growing old together?

    ☐ Yes ☐ No

19. How do you show each other affection?

_____

_____

_____

20. Does your show of affection met the needs of your fiancé?

    ☐ Yes ☐ No

21. Is your fiancé kind, gentle & understanding? ☐ Yes ☐ No

22. Why do you think that may be?

    _____

    _____

    _____

    _____

    _____

23. Is your fiancé understanding of your family? ☐ Yes ☐ No

24. What is your education level?

    HS 2Y 4Y M PhD

25. What is your fiancés education level?

    HS 2Y 4Y M PhD

26. Does your level of education bother you?

   ☐ Yes   ☐ No

27. If yes, explain

   _____

   _____

   _____

28. Does your fiancés level of education bother you?

   ☐ Yes   ☐ No

29. If yes, explain

   _____

   _____

   _____

30. Why are you attracted to your fiancé?

   _____

   _____

   _____

   _____

   _____

31. Why is your fiancé attracted to you?

_____

_____

_____

_____

_____

_____

_____

_____

_____

_____

32. What would you change about your fiancé?

_____

_____

_____

33. What would your fiancé change about you?

_____

_____

_____

_____

_____

_____

_____

After you have shared your answers:

1. What did you learn about your fiancé?

_____

_____

_____

_____

_____

_____

_____

_____

_____

_____

_____

_____

_____

_____

_____

_____

_____

2. What did you learn about yourself?

_____

_____

_____

_____

_____

_____

_____

_____

_____

_____

_____

_____

_____

_____

_____

_____

"For I know the plans I have for you,"

declares the LORD,

"plans to prosper you and not to harm you,

plans to give you hope and a future."

JER 29:11

FINANCES

Taking a moment to sit down and discuss the money matters of your future home and personal lives is an important step in keeping your marriage on track and harmonious. Other than communication, money is one of the top marriage stressors.

1. Who will be the primary financial provider in the family?
   HIM   HER

2. How will you decide on what major purchases to make?

   _____

   _____

   _____

   _____

3. Do you support your fiancé's career?   □ Yes   □ No

4. Will the wife work outside of the home?   □ Yes □ No

5. Who will pay the bill?   HIM   HER

6. Who will keep the checkbook?

    HIM   HER   BOTH

7. Will you tithe or support a local church?   □ Yes □ No

8. What is your philosophy on giving to charitable

    organizations?

    _____

    _____

    _____

    _____

    _____

9. How do you feel about the use of credit cards?

    _____

    _____

    _____

22

10. If either you or your spouse lost your job, what budget items would you cut?

_____

_____

_____

11. Will you have joint savings and checking accounts?

□ Yes   □ No

12. Will you keep your personal account?   □ Yes   □ No

13. Have you created a family budget?   □ Yes   □ No

14. Have you created an "emergency or rainy day" fund?

□ Yes   □ No

15. What percentage of your income will go toward home, car, groceries, utilities etc?

_____

_____

_____

1. What did you learn about your fiancé?

_____

_____

_____

_____

_____

_____

_____

_____

_____

_____

_____

_____

_____

_____

2. What did you learn about yourself?

_____

_____

_____

_____

_____

_____

_____

_____

_____

_____

_____

_____

_____

_____

A wife of noble character who can find?

She is worth far more than rubies...

She gets up while it is still dark; she provides

food for her family...

She watches over the affairs of her household and

does not eat the bread of idleness...

Many women do noble things, but you surpass

them all.

PROV 31: 10,15,27,29

HOME

Home-Sweet-Home. Home is a place of refuge - a place of comfort at the end of a busy day. Home is where we form the traditions of a family and keep a culture alive. Home is where no person should be a stranger and everyone is loved equally.

How will your humble abode fair?

1. Where do you want to live and in what setting would you want to live *(city, suburb, house, condo, etc.)*?

   _____

   _____

   _____

2. What do you expect your standard of living to be like after one year?

   _____

   _____

3. What to you expect your standard of living to be like after five years?

_____

_____

_____

_____

4. How will it affect you if it has not lived up to your expectations?

_____

_____

_____

_____

_____

5. How soon after you are married, do you expect to have your home reasonably furnished?

_____

_____

_____

6. Do you expect to change your furnishings to meet the house & home trend *(stay modern or up to speed)*?

_____

_____

_____

7. Will you do your own home maintenance? ☐ Yes ☐ No

8. Who will do the gardening/landscaping?

HE   SHE   BOTH

1. What did you learn about your fiancé?

_____

_____

_____

_____

_____

_____

_____

_____

_____

_____

_____

_____

_____

_____

_____

_____

2. What did you learn about yourself?

_____

_____

_____

_____

_____

_____

_____

_____

_____

_____

_____

_____

_____

_____

_____

_____

HOUSEKEEPING

Maid service or DIY, the housework must be done. Figure out what will work out best for your household. Traditional or modern couple – what's your style?

1. What type of food will you eat and who will prepare each meal?

   _____

   _____

   _____

   _____

2. How often will you eat out?

   _____

   _____

3. Who will pay for the meals when eating out?

   HE   SHE   BOTH

4. Who will do the laundry and ironing?

   HE SHE BOTH

5. Who will purchase groceries?

   HE   SHE BOTH

6. Who will make sure car maintenance is done?

   HE   SHE

7. Who will do general household cleaning and bed making?

   HE SHE

8. Who will wash and dry the dishes?

   HE   SHE BOTH

9. Do you want a pet in the home? If so, what type?

   _____

   _____

   _____

1. What did you learn about your fiancé?

_____

_____

_____

_____

_____

_____

_____

_____

_____

_____

_____

_____

_____

_____

_____

_____

2. What did you learn about yourself?

_____

_____

_____

_____

_____

_____

_____

_____

_____

_____

_____

_____

_____

_____

_____

_____

Your wife shall be like a fruitful vine

In the very heart of your house,

Your children like olive plants

All around your table.

Psalms 128:3 NKJV

CHILDREN AND PARENTING

With so many people concentrating on their careers first, children may not be on your immediate to do list. Maybe you have already had children and you wish to merge your 2 families – no matter the situation, discuss what you think your style of parenting is, or could be.

1. What is your attitude towards children?

    _____

    _____

    _____

    _____

2. When will you begin planning for children?

    _____

    _____

    _____

3. How many children do you wish to have?

_____

4. Have any children been lost due to death? ☐ Yes ☐ No

5. If yes – how long ago and how are you dealing with it now?

_____

_____

_____

_____

_____

_____

_____

_____

6. What would you do if you cannot conceive children of your own? Does your fiancé feel the same?

_____

_____

_____

_____

_____

_____

7. Are you Pro Life or Pro Choice?

LIFE   CHOICE

8. What is your view on birth control?

_____

_____

_____

_____

_____

9. What is your fiancé view on birth control?

_____

_____

_____

10. Who will be the primary caregiver for your children?

SHE   HE

11. How will you discipline them?

_____

_____

_____

_____

12. Who will be the primary disciplinarian?   SHE   HE

13. Will your children do chores?   □ Yes   □ No

14. At what age will they start doing chores?

_____

15. Will your children receive an allowance, if so, how much and how often?

_____

_____

16. If there are children from a previous marriage, will they live with you, how will they affect your day to day life?

_____

_____

_____

_____

_____

17. How will you deal with issues at their school?

_____

_____

_____

_____

_____

18. Do you get along with the other parent, if not, how will you deal with them regarding the children?

_____

_____

_____

_____

_____

_____

_____

19. Will any children from a previous marriage call you Mom and Dad or any special name, if not why?

_____

_____

_____

_____

_____

_____

_____

_____

1. What did you learn about your fiancé?

_____

_____

_____

_____

_____

_____

_____

_____

_____

_____

_____

_____

_____

_____

2. What did you learn about yourself?

_____

_____

_____

_____

_____

_____

_____

_____

_____

_____

_____

_____

_____

_____

_____

_____

The grace of the Lord Jesus Christ,

and the love of God,

and the communion of the Holy Spirit

be with you all.

Amen.

2 COR 12:14 NKJV

SOCIAL ACTIVITIES/CHURCH

Having a social life is very important to many people.
Being able to entertain in one's home by sharing
good times with friends is more than just something
that you like to do, it is a requirement.

Going to Church or a house of worship is the key
location for others.   Being around like-minded
individuals – *believers of your faith* – is not an option
for you it is a must.   Going to church every Sunday
morning and praise team/choir rehearsal is the
highlight of your Wednesday night.   What if your
fiancé doesn't feel the same way? How will you deal
with that?

1. Do you share the same beliefs; are you the same faith?

   □ Yes □ No

2. Do you attend the same house of worship? □ Yes □ No

3. Will you attend the same house of worship? □ Yes □ No

4. What will you teach your children regarding your faith?

   _____

   _____

   _____

   _____

   _____

5. Will you continue your hobbies once you are married?

   □ Yes □ No

6. Will you continue the same recreational activities?

   □ Yes □ No

7. Will you purse new hobbies or recreational activities once you are married, if so, individually, together and how often?

_____

_____

8. Are you willing to participate in activities solely to please your mate? □ Yes □ No

9. How will your personal friendships (his/her friends) change after marriage?

_____

_____

_____

_____

10. How do you feel about alcoholic beverages, smoking and guns in your home?

_____

_____

11. Where will you spend the holidays, birthdays and

anniversaries?

_____

_____

_____

12. Will you have certain times to spend with your friends?

□ Yes   □ No

13. Will you be joining any social clubs?   □ Yes   □ No

1. What did you learn about your fiancé?

_____

_____

_____

_____

_____

_____

_____

_____

_____

_____

_____

_____

_____

_____

2. What did you learn about yourself?

_____

_____

_____

_____

_____

_____

_____

_____

_____

_____

_____

_____

_____

_____

_____

_____

Let us discern for ourselves what is right;

let us learn together what is good.

Job 34:4

RED FLAGS

The questions listed below, should be thoroughly read and answered. If you feel uncomfortable about doing this section with your fiancé around, then choose to do this section during your meditation/prayer/quite time.

So many times our friends and family members will try to pull our coat tails to the "clues" that there is something just not good about a person. Many times we shrug it off and continue about our way. Then something happens and we say I should have seen it coming. Will, this is your moment to read with 20/20 vision and answer with a truthful heart. Don't think that if you answer in a positive fashion to a negative question that it will make that issue go away – it will not.

If you feel that you need assistance from a professional, please listen to your spirit and do so.

This does not mean that you no longer love your fiancé, it only means that you wish to have another set of eyes and ears to assist with a few concerns.

1. Does your fiancé seem to be irrationally jealous of friends, family or past relationships?   □ Yes   □ No

2. Is your fiancé prone to extreme emotional outbursts and/or very bad mood swings?   □ Yes   □ No

3. Does your fiancé displays controlling behavior?

   □ Yes   □ No

4. Is your fiancé unable to hold a job for any length of time?

   □ Yes   □ No

5. Are you and your fiancé unable to resolve your conflict?

   □ Yes   □ No

6. Does your fiancé exhibits dishonesty all the time?

   □ Yes   □ No

7. Does your fiancé treat you with respect?   □ Yes   □ No

8. Does your fiancé like to humiliate you in public?

   □ Yes   □ No

9. Does your fiancé like to gossip or tell untrue stories about your relationship? □ Yes   □ No

10. Is your fiancé overly dependent on others for money?

    □ Yes   □ No

11. Does your fiancé exhibits patterns of physical, emotional or sexual abuse towards you or others?

    □ Yes   □ No

12. Does your fiancé display signs of drug or alcohol abuse?

    □ Yes   □ No

Note: If any of these signs exist, and you are concerned about them, you should schedule a time to talk with a minister or counselor immediately.

After you have shared your answers:

1. What did you learn about your fiancé?

_____

_____

_____

_____

_____

_____

_____

_____

_____

_____

_____

_____

_____

_____

_____

2. What did you learn about yourself?

_____

_____

_____

_____

_____

_____

_____

_____

_____

_____

_____

_____

_____

_____

_____

_____

NOTES

NOTES

NOTES

NOTES

NOTES

LINKS

Links

www.blessingsallaround.com

www.angelachesterministries.org

www.blogtalkradio.com/I-Do-Radio

www.amazon.com

www.myspace.com/amilliongfx

AUTHOR

Rev. Angela Butts Chester, DD, is a pioneer in the field of family destiny fulfillment. With a passion for counseling, she blends her motivational spirit and a love for helping others, into a system that shows families how to keep the happiness, love, prosperity and abundance within the household.

Following in her family's footsteps, she became an ordained nondenominational minister in 2005. Starting a family ministry was a must for Rev. Chester, so Blessings All Around was created. This blessing ministry not only focuses on marrying couples, but various ceremonies that form bonds and traditions; ways to keep the family together.

Knowing that statistics speak against successful marriages, Rev. Chester has taken her expertise to the

Internet. As the host of I Do Radio, she discusses wedding issues to assist engaged couples with ceremony dos-and-don'ts and wedding vendor issues. Founder and President of the National Association of Black Wedding Officiants (NABWO), Rev. Chester, works with other ministers who know the importance of family in today's society.

As the author of **"Before You Tie The Knot"**, Angela Chester Ministries, focuses on keeping you on track and faith focused. Offering books, CDs and inspirational items to help keep you on the higher path, there is something for everyone at every stage of life.

Rev. Chester, is also a contributing author on "Life With Grace" by Rev. Paula Webb, with the inspirational story Morning Tea.